Slim for Life Secrets

SUSAN DAWSON-COOK, M.S.

Slim for Life Secrets
Copyright
© 2023 Susan Dawson-Cook
Published by Corazon del Oro
Communications, LLC
Cover Art by Pro DesignX
ISBN: 9798386314644

DISCLAIMER

This book offers ideas on how to improve fitness, lose weight and eat healthier. The content provided in this book is offered for informational purposes and should not be considered as medical advice, diagnosis, or treatment. Please consult with your physician before starting an exercise program. Please talk with your doctor before making dietary changes to ensure they are suitable for your current health status.

INTRODUCTION

Most people gravitate toward weight-loss plans they perceive will be easy. But no one loses weight or achieves any significant goal without commitment and hard work.

Although my Slim for Life tips may be difficult to follow at first, the good news is that once you make them a habit, they will be part of your lifestyle and will feel easy to continue. And the results you'll gain—more energy, joy, health, and an optimal body weight—will motivate you to continue with these new lifestyle habits for many years to come.

Over the course of my 30 years employed as a fitness professional, I trained hundreds of clients at an active adult community and a world-renowned spa. I've witnessed the transformation of dozens of lives. Many of the people I trained and taught in classes are over 50 and learned that it wasn't too late to make positive changes and live a better life.

If you would like additional resources, I also wrote *Fitter Than Ever at 40 and Beyond* and *Fitter Than Ever at 50 and Beyond* to help people succeed in making positive changes and transforming their lives. These books offer detailed information on how to start and maintain a safe exercise program and track heart rate (or perceived exertion) and Body Mass Index (BMI), how to improve the quality of your diet, how to identify roadblocks that are impeding your progress, and ways you can live a more mindful life.

I also offer Zoom yoga classes online and teach classes and retreats in San Carlos, Mexico. If you'd like to subscribe to my newsletter, you can do so using this landing page https://mailchi.mp/8113fa38f7ec/susans-zoom-yoga-classes

SLIM FOR LIFE SECRET #1
Avoid Binging at Parties

Curbing snack attacks and warding off the temptation to overeat at parties can be challenging. A small pre-event snack can stabilize blood sugar, keep energy levels high, and prevent intense hunger that can lead to binge eating. Increasing fat intake at meals will reduce hunger and possibly the need for snacks altogether.

The best snacks are filling and packed with nutrients. The worst ones are simple carbohydrates such as candy and pastries loaded with white sugar or corn syrup. Such treats give you a temporary blood sugar high followed by a sudden plummet, which lingers until you pop more sugar in your mouth.

Some of my favorite healthy snacks are small slices of cheese, a dozen nuts (almonds, pistachios or pecans are my favorites), and plain yogurt. You might have to experiment to see which snacks best help you get through vulnerable situations without a binge. Since I no longer snack and I avoid sugar (which always caused my worst cravings), binge eating for me has become a thing of the past.

Eating a small, filling snack ahead of time will allow you to make wiser food choices once you get to the party. Walk by the food table and decide what you're going to put on your plate first. Then get in line and serve yourself what you planned to eat. Savor your food. Once you finish, get rid of your plate, and talk to people some distance away from the food so you're not tempted to nibble.

Aim to drink in moderation. Alcoholic beverages are empty calories, which deplete rather than nourish your body. They also reduce inhibitions, leading to overeating. I know a geologist who lost 30 pounds in three months simply because he was assigned work at a "dry" mining camp (one where no alcohol was allowed).

If you must drink, alternate back and forth between your alcoholic beverage and club soda to reduce calorie consumption and the effects of the alcohol on your will power.

Stand, fidget, and dance. These "activities" burn calories. Standing burns more calories than sitting. A survey of career women established that those who sat for 361 minutes or more during an average workday were 1.7 times more likely to be overweight than those who sat for 30 minutes or less. Whether you're working or retired, aim to stay on your feet as much as possible. Sitting for long periods of time isn't just a diet buster: it has been linked to many health problems.

If possible, find an ally at the party who wants to employ similar mindful eating strategies. Then you can bond together and "just say no" each time the caterer waves yet another tempting tray in front of your nose.

When hosting a party, serve plenty of healthy, low-fat, low-calorie foods. Vegetable trays with low-fat dressing, fruit trays, cheese trays, and whole grain breadsticks are great options. Many of your guests will appreciate your efforts to provide healthy foods.

SLIM FOR LIFE SECRET #2
Travel (for Work or Pleasure) Without Gaining Weight

Sixteen years ago, while employed as a sales manager for an assistive technology company, I traveled to conferences and schools in many different states. Diet and exercise became a challenge, but within weeks, I had formulated a strategy. I found ways to exercise daily (even if in small bouts) and avoid sugar-laden breakfasts and unhealthy restaurants.

Aim to find hotels with gyms or near a place (indoor or outdoor) where you can exercise. Some hotels offer strength training tools you can check out to use in your room such as dumbbells or stability balls. One tool I highly recommend for travel is the TRX suspension trainer. It is great for strengthening major muscle groups as well as your core. If you're traveling overseas, you'll be able to use it any place you have a door!

Go   to https://store.trxtraining.com/shop/suspensio n-trainers/ to order a TRX trainer. I have written many articles with descriptions and photos of TRX exercises. Most of these are listed on the publication page of my fit women rock website http://fitwomenrock.com/?page_id=392

When traveling for work, I soon learned that restaurant meals posed the biggest threat to my plan to avoid weight gain. I worked hard to ward off the potential damage. The good news is that it's much easier to eat healthy on the run today than it was fifteen years ago. Many fast or to-go style restaurants now offer very healthy and/or low-calorie fare; but you must choose wisely.

To keep my eating in check, I traveled with plain (not sweetened) oatmeal packets, nuts, and tea bags. That way, I could breakfast in my hotel room, have more time to exercise, and leave feeling satisfied and ready to work. Eating ahead of time kept me from being tempted by doughnuts and sweet rolls, the usual "breakfast" offered at most of the conferences. A breakfast high in simple carbohydrates is not only a disaster for steady blood sugar and energy levels, it also drags you down even more when you're traveling and changing time zones.

I went for salads (dressing on the side), soups (tend to fill me up more than other foods), lunch-sized portions, and heart-healthy meals as often as possible. I sought restaurants offering lunch sized portions at dinner and ordered nutritious meals relatively low in calories (salads packed with fresh veggies and cheese—not processed meat—with dressing on the side); salmon or other fish filets - grilled or poached, not fried, and served with vegetables; grilled chicken, and some Asian and Mediterranean dishes).

I recommend searching for restaurant menus online before dining. Decide what you will order ahead of time based on calories and other nutritional information. I still do this often when I'm about to go out. This way you won't be tempted to order something with twice the calories while you're engaged in conversation or aren't feeling disciplined enough to make a thoughtful choice.

In my *Fitter Than Ever at 40 and Beyond* book, I included a top 10 *Health* article list of the healthiest fast-food restaurants. The link to that list is no longer online. I found another one but found it less than impressive. Foods in general weren't healthy and seemed very high in calories. For that reason, I decided to compile my own list based on my own experience and viewing different fast-food menus. I am not going to rank them, but I will offer my honest opinion on strengths and weaknesses.

Chipotle Mexican Grill specializes in tacos and burritos — a great option if you love healthy Mexican food. They also offer salads and quesadillas. This restaurant is one of my go-to places after swim meets. I find the portions too large, but the food is super delicious. The company buys mostly organic produce that is locally purchased and hormone- and antibiotic-free meats. Vegan and vegetarian options are also available and if you eat gluten free you can eat your burrito contents from a bowl, instead of wrapped in a tortilla (burrito bowl). Adding cheese and sour cream can up the calories quickly. Calories of different combos can be calculated at https://chipotle.com/nutrition-calculator

Another favorite of mine is In-N-Out Burger. We always stop at a Tucson location when we return from Mexico and don't have any food in the fridge. Since I don't eat gluten, I order the double-double cheeseburger, protein style (520 calories). The burger is wrapped in lettuce (and a thin layer of paper to make it easier to eat) instead of coming with a bun. The hamburger is 100 percent USDA ground chuck, free of additives, fillers, or preservatives. French fries are made with fresh potatoes (I've seen them machine dicing them). The burgers and fries are all high in sodium, but they have a very simple menu without a lot of elaborate, calorie laden options—a big benefit. Their menu with nutritional information can be found here https://www.in-n-out.com/menu/nutrition-info

Subway is a good lunch-on-the-go option to control calories if you're able to stick to eating a 6-inch sub. Bread is made fresh daily.

Comprehensive nutrition information is available at https://www.subway.com/en-US/MenuNutrition/Nutrition/NutritionGrid It was unclear to me on this nutrition page if calories listed are for 6- or 12-inch subs. I cut out processed meats (which increase cancer risk and are high in additives, including MSG), so I no longer buy sandwiches from this chain.

Wendy's is the third-largest hamburger fast food chain in the world. Their buns are loaded with preservatives. Burgers and fries are high in sodium. They do offer some nutritious salads https://order.wendys.com/category/102/freshmade-salads

With a proliferation of sushi restaurants in the US, most people can grab sushi in their neighborhood or wherever they're vacationing. Sushi is basically a seaweed wrap, usually with fish and rice inside and with soy sauce, pickled ginger, and wasabi handy to add for flavor. For many years, we dined in a neighborhood sushi restaurant almost every Friday.

Sushi is low in fat. Fish is rich in protein and loaded with heart healthy Omega-3 fatty acids. Sushi restaurants often serve other options that aren't so healthy (very high in saturated fat and sodium) and would be best to pass on, such as teriyaki bowls and fried noodles. Sushi made with raw fish puts you at risk for infection from bacteria or parasites. It is safer to opt for vegetarian sushi or sushi made with cooked fish.

Fast food places I tend to avoid are McDonald's, Arby's, Taco Bell, and Long John Silver's. In general, I recommend that you avoid places that offer super caloric foods you can't resist, that have no healthy options, or that don't list calories on their menu pages.

When traveling, especially for an extended time, your diet choices are critical. It's easy to swallow 1500 to 2000 calories in one poorly chosen restaurant meal. If you make good food choices, burning calories with exercise can be a second way to mitigate weight gain when traveling. Regular activity can also help manage stress, which is a common trigger for eating binges.

Here's what I did to stay active during my work-related trips:

1 - I chose hotels with gyms and pools (and verified they were open during the hours I could use them). Some hotels also offer free use of nearby fitness facilities. This can be great if they're conveniently located.

2 - I awoke early every morning to exercise. Since I was on my feet most of the day, I chose swimming or stationary bicycling for aerobic exercise. I only had time for about 30 minutes of exercise daily, but I was able to work in additional short bursts of activity. If you're going to be sitting most of the day, the treadmill and/or the elliptical will be good choices if no

physical limitations make those activities prohibitive.

3 - I walked whenever possible — up and down the hall or around the parking lot or block during lunches and breaks between meetings and around the airport terminal when waiting for flights. I took the stairs to get to my hotel room when I had an upper-level floor. Any time you can insert a few minutes of activity, do so!

4 - I put a resistance band around my ankles when getting ready in the morning. Moving around the room like this with the bands helped tone my thighs and buttocks.

When planning leisure travel, I often dive into activities I don't normally do at home. I swim in a new body of water (ocean or lake), practice yoga (outdoors, of course), rent an e-bike, and take long hikes or walks.

Sometimes, we embark on activity-based vacations. So far, my husband and I have gone scuba diving in Mexico, Belize, Jamaica, the

Bahamas, and Costa Rica, cycled through the Swiss Alps, hiked to Machu Picchu, circumnavigated several Greek Islands in the Ionian Sea, and hiked to many Mayan Ruins in Belize and Guatemala. All these trips were delightful fun. While staying active all day, we met interesting people from around the world and enjoyed beautiful views and plenty of fresh air! What could be better?

SLIM FOR LIFE SECRET #3
Minimize Restaurant Meals

It's understandable that you might need to eat out when you're traveling, but what do you do when you're in town? If you're dining out two or more nights a week, please reconsider this habit. It will greatly simplify and ease your journey to wellness.

Did you know that many restaurant meals are packed with 2000 or more calories? It's true. And that's just for the appetizer, soup or salad, main course, and dessert. That doesn't even include your glass or two of wine or the fancy cocktail you decide to order. In a book entitled,

So You're Fat. Now What? cardiologist Salvatore Tirrito says, "I will go as far to say that if you eat out more than twice a week, you are probably never going to lose any weight."

Honestly, his assessment corresponds with what I've observed after more than thirty years on the ground training and teaching fitness. I never trained a client who wanted to lose weight, ate out more than three times a week and reached their weight loss goal. It is like trying to swim upstream in a heavy current!

I suggest you save yourself the needless frustration. Whenever you eat out, you force yourself to cope with serious temptation that most of us find difficult to overcome. Choosing a salad or heart-health dish will be difficult when your friends are ordering pizza or 16 oz. steaks.

Until you reach your goal weight, please keep meals out to a minimum and when you do eat out, choose restaurants that list calories of menu items and that serve smaller portions. Eating in restaurants these days essentially teaches you to not be satisfied until you've finished enormous quantities of food!

Do you want to know how many calories (and how much saturated fat, etc.) you consume when you eat out? Go to restaurant websites to learn the ugly truth.

Many of these links change often, so if you get a dead link, go to the main website, and then hunt around. Some sites only have nutrition listed if you click a link next to each item; others have a page that lists nutritional information on all available items.

I have decided not to list links in this book since the menus and links change so often. It's easy enough to search on your phone before you go. If a restaurant doesn't share nutritional information, it's best to stay away.

These snacks and meals can really blow your diet…

- Starbucks Grande Café Vanilla Frappuccino with blueberry muffin **910 calories**
- Pizza Hut personal pan cheese pizza and 16-oz. Coke **830 calories**
- Ben and Jerry's Chunky Monkey (1 pint) **1160 calories**
- Schlotzsky's Deli Original Sandwich and 16-oz Coke **975 calories**
- Big Mac, medium fries, and chocolate shake at McDonald's **1470 calories**

Any time nutrition information isn't available, assume you are getting 600 calories from each appetizer, 400 for a soup or salad, 1000 for a main course and 600 for a dessert.

Can you say "Ouch?" Are you still too speechless? Let me say it for you—"Ouch!" If you study restaurant menus too long, you might need to have the paramedics standing by. The shock factor is so extreme.

The quickest way to resuscitate your diet is to take control and eat more meals at home. I intentionally minimize meals out for better health and weight control. I like to have control over what I'm eating and to avoid foods with added sugar or trans fat. I can consume fewer calories and healthier meals eating at home and save a lot of money, too.

SLIM FOR LIFE SECRET #4
Avoid Fake Food (or Just Eat Real Food)

If you've ever read food labels, you'll notice that many items contain more than 10 ingredients. Those "fresh" baked items from the grocery store may contain 25 or 30 ingredients, including many preservatives—so the bread or pastry can stay on the shelf longer without spoiling—and colorants to make the food look tasty so it will lure you to buy it. There are likely some unhealthy oils thrown into the mix.

A Dairy Queen chocolate ice cream cone contains 22 ingredients. I bet most people aren't aware of this. Many Americans consume five pounds of additives per year. Yuck! I read labels like that and think that item doesn't sound at all like food to me! And I don't buy it.

One of the big risks of eating preservative-rich foods is that many are classified as hyperpalatable. What this means is that food companies have designed them to tap into your brain's reward system, predisposing you and all the rest of us to have an addictive-like craving for them.

If we eat enough of these foods, eventually whole foods (that are not processed at all or that are minimally processed) will begin to taste bland and inedible and only unhealthy foods packed with salt, sugar, and/or fat will do. Once addictive behavior takes hold, it is much harder for a person to eat to sate hunger instead of giving into emotional cravings.

Lab rats given unlimited access to a diet high in carbohydrates and fat will nearly eat themselves to death and will walk across an electrified plate to get to their junk food. Once addicted to all three substances, when given a choice between sugar, cocaine and alcohol, the rats ran straight for the sugar.

If you have been suffering under a shroud of guilt, thinking that it's your fault that you have no will power to stop eating this stuff, recognize that food companies are manipulating minds (and tastebuds) so almost no one who eats this stuff can say *no*. The only way to free yourself is to stop eating this addictive food.

When you constantly indulge in foods rich in sugar and fat, overeating and addiction becomes part of your gene expression. Altering your genetic "story" starts that first day you choose to eat an apple instead of a candy bar.

I'm very familiar with food addiction because I suffered from it for years. There were times where the only thing that mattered was sinking my teeth into a pizza with melted cheese or getting my hands on that bag of vending machine chocolates (that had fallen from the hook and gotten stuck on the way down)! I wouldn't have cared if our dormitory roof collapsed, or the fire alarm went off. My hands literally trembled when I was in line waiting to buy junk food at a convenience store.

From my experience, the only path to freedom is to wean yourself off these foods. They wreak havoc on your weight, your self-esteem, and your health.

No one really knows the long-term effects of eating a preservative-rich diet. I have read studies that show that if certain food particles, such as the artificial sweetener sucralose, are not recognized by the digestive system, they may remain in your gut. Some preservatives upset the natural balance of intestinal flora. Is there any wonder most Americans never leave home without several different products for upset stomachs and bowel issues?

If you experience headaches or other symptoms from MSG, be aware that more than 40 different items with different names also contain this harmful substance including seemingly benign items such as gelatin and whey protein. "Spices" can include almost anything.

That's why when grilling fish or any other meat, I mix up my own blend of healthy spices instead of opting for a pre-made spice mix that is full of questionable ingredients. It only takes a minute.

In general, shop the perimeter of the grocery store. That's where you'll usually find the "real" food. Even then, please read labels like a hawk. You'll be shocked by what you learn—so many foods we buy on autopilot such as spaghetti sauce, salad dressings, and even artificial meats include sugar or high fructose corn syrup. I prefer to instead buy organic tomato sauce or diced tomatoes, Primal Kitchen salad dressings, and small quantities of (mostly organic) meat.

I also buy fresh (mostly organic) fruits and vegetables, meat, dairy, lentils, quinoa, coffee, and tea. If you've been skimping on produce purchases because of budget, re-evaluate. Do you want to invest money now feeding your body nutritious food to stay healthy or pay it to the hospital later after your body has broken down due to poor nutrition?

Some of my favorite foods are grilled salmon, bonita (a fish my neighbors catch in Mexico), chicken, ribeye steak, mushrooms sauteed in olive oil, fresh yogurt (I make it myself), berries of any kind (blackberries, blueberries, strawberries, etc.), grapes, nuts (pistachios, pecans, macadamia nuts), spinach, asparagus, avocados, kale, tomatoes, cucumber, broccoli, cheese (Swiss, feta, and Manchego) and sweet potatoes. Whenever possible, I buy organic.

SLIM FOR LIFE SECRET #5
Ditch Caloric Beverages

When my daughter was in high school, she lost 20 pounds. She didn't try a starvation diet. She didn't cut out all dairy or eat only soup. She didn't change what she ate at all in fact. She simply stopped drinking juice and soda.

A glass of liquids other than water or black tea or coffee usually means beaucoup calories. You can drink a whole day's worth of calories inadvertently in a matter of minutes. A single soda contains about 200 calories. That doesn't sound like much, but if you drink three sodas and two glasses of juice during the day, you'll top 1000 calories with drinks alone.

Sodas and energy drinks contain harmful chemicals and incite hunger due to their high sugar content. Diet drinks are as bad or worse as sugar-laden ones, sporting a long ingredient list of chemicals. Aspartame (Nutrasweet, Equal and others) and Sucralose (Splenda and others) have possible links to cancer and neurological disease. Both artificial sweeteners have been linked to weight gain.

Workout or electrolyte drinks, such as Gatorade (127 calories for 16 oz.), that are high in sugar, may compromise dental health. I have had consistently clean dental checkups since I ditched the habit of drinking sugary energy drinks at work. Low calorie workout drinks tend to be loaded with artificial sweeteners and other chemicals.

I drink water with a dose of salt and magnesium whenever I need electrolytes. A reliable electrolyte supplement you can take after long workouts or exercising in the heat is Hi-Lyte, which offers sodium, potassium and magnesium without any added sugar or chemicals.

Alcoholic beverages can be another caloric black hole. A four-ounce margarita packs about 168 calories, but depending on the size of your drink glass, you might get double or triple the calories. Some drinks excessively high in calories are strawberry daiquiris, piña coladas, and Long Island iced tea (780 calories).

The spiritual path I'm following today precludes the consumption of alcohol. But I do recall how drinking a beer or glass of wine at parties (when there was a long wait for food) took the edge off my appetite and helped me to relax, enabling me to eat less.

I suggest drinking water, unsweetened coffee and tea and having a soda or an alcoholic drink only occasionally. If plain water frustrates your taste buds, try squeezing in a few drops of lemon juice or adding a tablespoon of coconut water. By dumping the caloric drink habit, you will likely lose weight if you don't subconsciously (or consciously) decide to "reward" yourself with more food.

SLIM FOR LIFE SECRET #6
Avoid Artificial Sweeteners

Consuming foods and beverages with artificial sweeteners might seem like the perfect way to kick your weight loss plan into high gear. They contain fewer calories than sugar-laden drinks and will lead to weight loss, right?

Think again. The research shows just the opposite. People who consume artificial sweeteners tend to weigh more than those who turn their noses up at them.

Artificial sweeteners are simple carbohydrates that don't provide the body with any nutrients yet cause elevated blood sugar levels.

Read your labels. Drinks and foods containing aspartame will not only sabotage your weight loss efforts, they may also sabotage your health. Aspartame, made by joining the amino acids aspartic acid and phenylalanine, although declared safe by many certifying agencies, possibly negatively impacts health.

It is purportedly 200 times as sweet as sugar, meaning you could use a much smaller quantity and still be satisfied, which once again sounds good, but isn't so great when you dig deeper.

Many studies indicate consuming artificial sweeteners correlates with weight gain. For some reason, rats and people consuming artificial sweeteners ate up to four times as much as people and rats eating only foods sweetened with regular sugar! It appears that consuming artificial sweeteners interferes somehow with the body's natural ability to regulate calorie intake.

A study following thousands of residents of San Antonio for 10 years found those who drank more than 21 servings of diet drinks a week were at twice the risk of becoming overweight or obese, and the more diet soda people drank, the greater the risk.

Another study found that participants drinking diet soda had a 70 percent greater increase in waist size over a 10-year period compared to non-diet soda drinkers. Those who drank two or more diet sodas a day had a 500 percent greater increase in waist size.

Research published in the *Journal of the Academy of Nutrition and Dietetics* indicated that people who drink diet beverages compensate for their "saved" calories by eating more foods high in sugar, sodium, and unhealthy fats.

I'll add some anecdotal evidence to this mix. During the only time in my life where I experienced weight problems (in college), I drank two or three diet sodas per day. I look back and remember how I felt constantly hungry and deprived. I even dreamed about fattening food at night! Somehow, artificial sweeteners had the same or even a worse effect on my cravings as actual sugar.

Sucralose, used in many beverages and even yogurt, is another commonly used artificial sweetener with questionable consequences on weight and health. I suggest you ditch the diet sodas and the "sugar-free" junk food and pour yourself a glass of water with a little lemon instead.

SLIM FOR LIFE SECRET #7
Eat Nutritious, Filling Foods

Many people who reduce caloric intake complain of rabid hunger. It's impossible to lose weight when you're constantly starving. I know because I've tried it.

Oh, I lost a few pounds here and there for a few days. Eventually, being the human I am and disliking the discomfort of a constantly growling stomach, I decided I didn't want to dream about food anymore and obsess about it all day...

So, I started eating. And once I started, since I was so starved (enough that I probably would have eaten wallpaper paste if that was all that was available), I ate and ate and ate!

By savoring satisfying, filling foods, you can lose weight without suffering from uncomfortable hunger pangs that inevitably lead to bingeing. Foods high in fat or fiber provide a sense of fullness that lasts. Increasing protein intake can also help with appetite control.

Foods high in sugar will raise and crash your blood sugar and lead you to crave food more often. I can reduce my food consumption by about 20 percent (easily) by cutting out sweets. A very good friend of mine lost eight pounds in one month simply by eliminating sugar!

I recently started eating yogurt for breakfast most mornings. I add melted butter, fruit, and nuts to balance it out. Yogurt is rich in calcium, B vitamins, and most contain probiotics, which can improve digestive health. Other hunger sating foods that I recommend are oatmeal, Swiss muesli, soups (homemade, not canned, packed with lentils, quinoa, pinto beans, and/or mung beans), toast with peanut or almond butter, and apples with peanut butter. Baked oatmeal with peaches and blueberries is also delicious.

If you decide to adopt my yogurt habit, don't think you have to kiss enjoyment of breakfast goodbye! A yogurt breakfast doesn't have to be boring. Add blueberries, raspberries, mango, flax seed, chia seeds, macadamia nuts, sliced banana, honey, raisins, or other dried fruit, and try seasoning with cinnamon or cardamom.

SLIM FOR LIFE SECRET #8
Stabilize Blood Sugar

If you experience headaches and/or mild dizziness when a meal comes late, and highs and lows in energy throughout the day, you likely have blood sugar issues.

Many people who haven't been diagnosed with diabetes experience blood sugar instability due to insulin resistance, where a high-carbohydrate eater's tired pancreas is unable to produce sufficient insulin to regulate blood sugar.

I experienced this in the past, largely because of decades of athletic training and being told I needed to eat often and load up on carbohydrates. The first red-flag I received was experiencing dizziness shortly after consuming pre-race energy gels. Some digging deeper led me to a new way of eating that is known as Low Carbohydrate High Fat (LCHF). Basically, my diet revolves around meat, dairy, fruits, and vegetables. I rarely consume grains and eat no sugar.

What is usually healthiest for most people — regardless of their activity level — is a diet free of sugar and relatively low in carbohydrates. Healthy carbohydrates can be found in vegetables, fruits, and legumes.

Many people can also benefit from intermittent fasting or time restricted eating (TRE), which involves a daily fast, usually of about 16 hours, which is cleansing for your digestive system and is purported to improve blood sugar and cholesterol levels as well as brain health.

Most fasters simply stop eating after dinner and then delay their breakfast until as late as possible the next day. For example, I usually eat dinner at 6 PM and have breakfast at 9 or 10 AM. Every day, I fast for a minimum of 15 hours and up to 20 hours.

Avoid restricting your calories too excessively (eating less than 1200 calories per day), though, because it may result in slowing of your metabolism, loss of muscle mass, and out-of-control hunger.

Most people lose weight (while eating satisfying meals) with time restricted eating for two main reasons.

First, this way of eating reduces the time where food is consumed.

Secondly, as your body adjusts to fasting, you will sometimes experience a state of ketosis (where fat, instead of sugar, is being used as fuel by the body) where hunger completely dissipates. Ketosis is amazing, really.

Sometimes I wake up not in ketosis and feel mildly hungry while I'm checking emails and surfing for news. Then I swim for an hour and move into ketosis and experience no hunger at all and can easily wait two or more hours post-workout to eat breakfast!

You can continue with time restricted eating if it is safe for you, and you have found success with it already. If you hadn't tried TRE before and want to try it, consult with your doctor first.

If this change to your way of eating is approved, you can start by moving your breakfast ahead or dinner back by one hour and as you get more comfortable, you can slowly widen your fasting window.

SLIM FOR LIFE SECRET #9
Avoid Dousing Food with Extra Calories

You can easily triple or more your calories by dousing your food with sauces, gravy, and/or too much salad dressing. Dumping a ton of sugar and cream into coffee is another choice most people make without thinking much about the exorbitant number of additional calories.

Consider using a low-cal salad dressing or using olive oil and vinegar instead of high-calorie dressings like Blue Cheese and Thousand Island. It is always best to avoid any salad dressing that includes inflammatory vegetable oils. Dressings made with avocado or olive oil are the healthiest.

Consider measuring the amount of sugar and cream you add to coffee and trying to gradually reduce how much you use. Learn to drizzle instead of douse food with sauces, gravy, and or dressings.

I've learned to enjoy the flavoring that seasonings provide. Some of my favorites are dill, cinnamon, cardamom, lemon grass, turmeric, basil, garlic, fennel seeds, and oregano. All have very few calories and add wonderful flavor to food. Many are also rich in antioxidants, which reduces inflammation in your body.

SLIM FOR LIFE SECRET #10
Eat Mindfully

Many of us develop the habit of reading, watching TV or working on the computer while eating. Maybe we sit down in front of the TV with a bag of chips only to find when the show ends or we're interrupted by an ad or our phone that we've polished off the whole bag! Mindless eating is a habit that is disastrous for your health and waistline.

If you're engaged in some other activity beyond eating, your mind and body don't fully process that you're enjoying a meal. Often the "full" feeling won't come as soon or ever. More than likely, you'll overeat a lot and barely notice. If you're holding a plate of food in your lap while watching TV, you may gobble it down quickly because you're focused on the show plot, not what you're shoveling into your mouth.

Normally, your stomach takes about 10 minutes to give you a signal that you're full but if you eat faster than that, you won't receive a signal in time. And if your mind is somewhere else, you won't ever get one.

Break the doing-something-else-while-eating habit and you'll find yourself consuming fewer calories at meals without feeling deprived. Always eat at your kitchen or dining room table. Engage in conversation or if you're alone, simply savor each bite of food.

Drink a glass of water before you begin eating (dehydration can sometimes be misinterpreted as hunger). Eat slowly and chew your food well before swallowing. Put your fork down often. This will not only improve digestion but will reduce your total food consumption. It takes several minutes for your stomach to "register" that it's full.

If possible, eat on a lunch plate (rather than a large dinner plate) so you are less tempted to serve yourself more food than needed to fill you up. Research has shown people eat less when using smaller plates and plates that have high contrast compared to the color of their food.

Meat servings should be no larger than your fist and 75 percent of your plate should be filled with fruits and vegetables. Don't force yourself to finish everything on the plate. Shun seconds unless you are still hungry. If you need to eat more to feel sated, serve yourself a second helping of broccoli over potatoes or more meat.

SLIM FOR LIFE SECRET #11
Choose Carbohydrates Wisely

Carbohydrates aren't necessarily bad. Many of them are healthy. What's important to note is that that certain members of this food group can lead to added pounds, health issues, and an out-of-control craving for more carbs.

Simple carbohydrates such as sugar, syrups, cakes, and cookies tend to digest quickly and increase appetite, whereas complex carbohydrates such as whole grain breads, legumes, vegetables, and lower carbohydrate fruits will improve your digestion and give you a sense of fullness and satiety that will last for hours.

Choose whole grain bread over white, whole grain pasta over white, wild rice over white, organic oatmeal over cold cereals laden with sugar and preservatives. Vegetables and fruits are also high in carbohydrates and should form the foundation of most peoples' diets.

"Starchy" carbohydrates such as white bread, pies, cookies, cakes, and crackers are loaded with fat and preservatives and provide scanty vitamins and minerals. These simple carbohydrates quickly assault your blood stream, raising blood sugar for a short period of time before you experience another sugar crash.

People who eat a lot of starchy carbohydrates tend to reflexively reach for more sugar whenever they experience a sugar crash. This is a vicious cycle that needs to be broken. Don't fall in the trap of buying a sugar-laden treat that is labeled "low-fat" or "organic." If sugar is high on the list of ingredients, buy something else.

Aim to replace all starchy carbohydrates with complex carbohydrates (whole grains). Oatmeal, whole grain breads, quinoa, and wild rice are some examples of complex carbohydrates.

If you're gluten intolerant, suffer from migraines, or have other digestive issues, you may want to consider eliminating most or all grains from your diet. The best way to test food intolerances is to eliminate a suspected food for a few weeks and see if you notice a change in your health or energy level.

SLIM FOR LIFE SECRET #12
Eliminate Emotional Eating

Stress can trigger over-eating and other bad habits such as shopping binges and drug and alcohol abuse. Dopamine, the "feel good" neurotransmitter, tends to be lowest in the late afternoon, making us crave a reward. Low dopamine and serotonin levels often compel people to eat anything in sight (especially foods high in sugar and fat).

This compulsion to eat too much of the wrong foods can be an addiction very similar to a frantic desire for drugs and alcohol. Late afternoon and evenings are times when many of us need to be armed and ready to combat this impulsive "I have to have it now" hunger with a healthy and satisfying snack.

It can be tempting to turn to food for solace when life gets difficult. Unfortunately, binging on too much or unhealthy food can lead to weight gain during times of trouble. If you are using food to soothe emotions and its wreaking havoc on your waistline, you can move toward replacing this habit with another behavior.

When I was a college student at Clemson, I'd go out on the weekends and indulge in way too many drinks for fun and to cope with the stress of college life. After a night out, my friends and I would polish off a large pizza within minutes because the alcohol had loosened our inhibitions. I'd try to return to dieting Monday morning but would end up rewarding myself with chips, popcorn, and sweets whenever it came time to study for a test or exam.

Feeling distressed over a breakup with a boyfriend or some other issue, I'd reach for more junk food. My diet rollercoaster and these emotional eating habits led to a weight gain of more than 25 pounds. That's quite a lot of weight for my small frame to carry!

I decided something had to change. I gradually introduced different ways of dealing with my emotional rollercoaster rides. Okay, so maybe I overdid it at first. I would go out and run until my legs threatened to give out underneath me.

Was that extreme? Yes. But it made me feel empowered. I've found writing to be another powerful outlet for stress and suffering. To this day, I tend to exercise, meditate, go to a quiet outdoor space, or write over grabbing a bag of chips whenever stress strikes. And there are no negative side effects either (weight gain, guilt, poor health).

It required hard work to establish new eating habits. I used to salivate just watching a food commercial on TV. Eating was an emotional reaction instead of a reaction to hunger. I became a food drama queen and allowed my brain to swindle me into believing I had to have food to endure this or that "horrible" period of stress.

My eating today is hunger driven. If pangs of hunger or stomach noises make it difficult to keep writing, I'll eat a meal. To keep on a comfortable schedule, I try not to vary my mealtimes by more than an hour.

When someone offers me food when I'm not hungry, I politely decline. Watching food commercials on TV never propels me toward the refrigerator unless it's close to mealtime. I'm not telling you this to brag. I'm doing this to encourage you. I've already told you enough stories about how far off track I once was to give you evidence that if I can do it, so can you!

If you learn to react to real hunger and not impulse on a regular basis it will start to become a habit and no longer a challenge of willpower. And then if you can find activities outside the realm of eating and drinking to cope with stress, you'll be well on your way to success!

We're all wired differently, so maybe you won't find the activities that feed my soul (exercise, yoga, writing, time outdoors) appropriate to put in place of your emotional eating habits. Use whatever activities you enjoy—so that you'll feel better (rather than guilty) afterward.

Maybe you can take a warm bath, play a musical instrument, paint or draw, read a good book, meditate, call a friend, get a massage or pedicure, do a Yoga Nidra session, or take a long walk. Even a five-minute time out for some long, restorative breaths will lower your stress level, blood pressure and heart rate. All of these are likely to release "feel good" hormones and won't leave you with a guilt hangover.

Once you begin assuaging your stress with non-food pleasures, eating will no longer be the automatic turn-to response when something goes wrong. And maybe that juicy burger you see on TV will no longer send you racing toward the refrigerator.

SLIM FOR LIFE SECRET #13
Mindful Grocery Shopping

We've all heard the *don't shop when you're hungry* suggestion before, but do you actually follow it? If not, please start today. Even the most disciplined person's willpower crumbles under the wrong circumstances.

If it has been hours since your last meal, pushing the shopping cart past baked goods and tempting foods at the deli without grabbing something (or a few somethings) will be nearly impossible. Since like you, I'm only human, I've ended up with unintended items because of this slip up.

Taking a list helps if you stick to it. Walking only the perimeter of the store is safest—all the junk lurks in the middle aisles. Remember, if the pastries, candy bars, and ice cream never make it to your house, they won't make it to your mouth...or your waistline. One of my biggest strategies for staying away from sweets is never buying them!

I know I mentioned this before, but I'm going to say it again because it's very important. If you don't want to spend time reading labels, please buy items that don't have an ingredient list—fresh food. That makes shopping super easy and doesn't require reading glasses. In the long run, it will improve your health and help you drop unwanted pounds.

People often complain that healthy food costs too much. This is just another excuse. If you buy and consume only real food—meat, fruits, vegetables, nuts, and dairy (no "healthy" snack foods, microwave dinners, packaged desserts and cereal)—you will find that your grocery bills will stay very reasonable. And your body will thank you for it!

SLIM FOR LIFE SECRET #14
Find Enjoyable Exercise

Most people don't enjoy doing the same workout day after day. If your cardio consists of walking mindlessly on the treadmill five days a week, you might get to the point where you'd rather get a root canal than endure yet another boring workout.

If you hate your chosen exercise modality or are bored with it, eventually you will quit. At the minimum, you'll make excuses not to do it. That's why you should take time early on to seek out exercise you enjoy. There are so many different modes of activity. Swimming, running, walking, hiking, tennis (and other racquet sports such as pickleball and ping pong), golf (walking the course), bicycling, stationary gym equipment, kayaking, paddle boarding, rappelling, dance (salsa, merengue, aerobic, ballroom, country, so many others), yoga, Pilates, drumming, and water aerobics.

Spend a month experimenting and then narrow down to what you like the most, so you keep moving. Most of you will find that mixing it up with two or more activities works best.

Nancy Patchell Knoll, a former SaddleBrooke, Arizona resident and client who followed my *Fitter Than Ever* program, wrote, "As a child, I sat inside reading and did well in school. I did not like playing outside and never played sports like other kids. I barely tolerated required PE courses and did the least possible."

By 2009, Nancy was in her 60s and her lifetime of inactivity had caught up with her. Nancy's doctor urged her to exercise, and she committed to trying my program for six months.

"My BMI and body fat analysis were horrifying. I had worn elastic waist, stretchy pants for decades so I had no idea that I was as big as I measured. I also realized I hadn't looked at myself in a full-length mirror for a long time and was relying on mirrors showing my top half only.

"The first exercise class I took just about killed me in the first three minutes. I was having trouble breathing and every muscle in my body hurt—and the class had barely begun. I realized how truly out of shape I was. Everyone told me things would get better as I got into shape, but I was still skeptical."

Jump ahead two months. "As I was able to do more and last longer, I started feeling a sense of pride in myself. An avowed couch potato having fun in aerobics class? Maybe I had changed."

Nancy continued exercising during her summer months away from SaddleBrooke. "I found two new-to-me exercises in Illinois that are social, fun, and great workouts. One is Nordic walking—I just bought my second set of poles to take back to Arizona. The other is the senior version of Drums Alive, which uses drumming as the exercise. Liking the exercise classes made it so much easier to go. For the first time in my life, exercise is a part of my day and my routine. I make time for it daily. On the few days I can't, it feels weird not to be doing something physical. I just bought two pairs of jeans with zippers and all!"

Consider your personality when you choose exercise modalities and then soon you, like Nancy, will have an exercise success story to tell. Some people really enjoy team activities. Others like to have their exercise be meditative or an outdoor nature experience. I tend to have days when I want to exercise alone and others where I want to be more social. I take/teach classes some days and do solo walks, kayaks, and swims other days. I love hiking in parks and on beaches where I feel connected to nature. In addition to exercise opportunities, I find these outdoor sessions relaxing and restorative.

Many people find a buddy system improves commitment and motivation to exercise. Your buddy can be someone (or more than one person) you exercise with and/or speak to periodically to provide and ask for encouragement along the way.

My 89-year-old mother—who has never enjoyed exercise--often walks with a neighbor shortly after awakening. Having a friend to lean on can be especially helpful when busy schedules and stressful life circumstances threaten to derail you from your program.

Most people work harder around others. Perhaps you can run or walk with friends who maintain a similar pace so you can socialize and push yourself at the same time. You could find out about bike rides or running groups in your community so you can meet and connect with others who enjoy the sport. You could join a U.S. Masters Swimming team (https://www.usms.org/clubs) and engage in organized interval swimming workouts instead of slogging out endless boring laps. Many other countries have competitive swimming groups and races available for adults.

SLIM FOR LIFE SECRET #15
Avoid Over-Exercising

You probably thought you would never hear me say don't exercise too much, but here I go...Don't exercise too much! I've done it before, and it only made my battle with weight more difficult. I felt so frustrated and angry that I was running so many miles and hating it and still wasn't losing weight. It took me a few years to learn why this happens.

Like a starvation diet, extreme levels of activity confuse the body and tend to make it hoard every calorie as if it might be your last. It may also incite the release of stress hormones, which makes it even more difficult to lose weight.

Many studies, including a review that followed *The Biggest Loser* contestants, show that RMR (resting metabolic rate) slows when people follow extreme exercise and diet plans. This makes weight loss and maintenance extremely difficult and frustrating!

I know dozens of overweight athletes who exercise for four or more hours per day and haven't lost weight. If your goal is to participate in long distance events, engage in a moderate amount of exercise until you achieve your goal weight and then gradually increase duration and intensity. Why not make things easier on yourself rather than as difficult as possible?

The best way to avoid a major decline in RMR is to take a moderate approach to caloric intake and exercise. You will have a much better chance of losing weight if you keep your exercise to 60 to 90 minutes per day. You can burn additional calories by sitting less. Moderate, rather than fanatical, exercise offers the most health benefits anyway.

If you want to compete in triathlons, sign up for the mini-triathlons (~800 yard swim, ~12 mile bike, 3 mile run), which give you a good balance of a moderate amount of the three activities.

SLIM FOR LIFE SECRET #16
Stay Busy

Many retirees gain weight. Retirees are often less busy than they were when working a full- or part-time job. With more available free time, thoughts tend to drift toward the next snack or meal. And the refrigerator is just a little too available.

If you find yourself struggling with weight gain or eating issues due to being at home, below are some strategies you can try to mitigate this issue:

- Seek a volunteer opportunity
- Join a book group

- Attend a class at a community college on a subject of interest
- Join a crafts or music group
- Go to the library or a park for a couple of hours daily to get out of the house

Another issue that clients have complained to me about is facing constant exposure to food when attending events. You go to a book club meeting and plates of cookies are waiting for you. You go to a knitting group and there's a platter of cheese and crackers tempting you. I recommend that you join (or start) groups that don't serve food between meals.

If you join groups where snacks are everywhere, you'll want to commit to not munching in advance.

SLIM FOR LIFE SECRET #17
Dump the Excuses

You won't succeed at losing weight or changing your habits until you commit to these efforts. There are generally five stages people go through before making major life changes.

These are pre-contemplation (not yet ready to change), contemplation (weighing the costs and benefits), preparation (buying a gym membership, hiring a personal trainer), action (exercising, eating healthy), and maintenance (healthy lifestyle has become a habit and is no longer a struggle). By the time you reach the preparation stage, you need to convince yourself that making excuses will no longer be acceptable.

Most of us conjure up excuses to avoid things we deem unpleasant. I tend to experience a variety of mysterious illnesses the day before dental appointments.

If you started following my Slim for Life Secret on enjoyable exercise, you should be engaging an activity you look forward to and enjoy and have no reason to try to avoid it! Hopefully, you've begun trying new food items and have begun to develop a taste for healthier fare.

Long before you picked up this book, you had already made a commitment to certain aspects of your life — non-negotiable responsibilities that you do daily no matter what.

If you're employed, you go to work every day unless you're ill or on vacation. Hopefully, you brush your teeth two or more times a day to maintain your dental health. If you're raising a family, you undoubtedly grocery shop and prepare balanced meals with help from your spouse. You don't make an excuse and say you're not fixing dinner one night, leaving everyone hungry!

You need to establish a mindset for healthy eating and exercise like your approach to brushing your teeth or fixing dinner or going to work or a doctor's appointment—that it is a responsibility, not something you shrug off with an "I don't have time today."

Pre-schedule your exercise sessions. Commit time to healthy eating today (buying healthy food items, looking up healthy recipes, and preparing food), instead of telling yourself that you will do it tomorrow or next week or next month.

Make healthy living a part of each day (even when you're on vacation) instead of making excuses that trap you in a rut. You're worth investing the effort.

Research shows that people tend to eat more when they think about how they'll diet tomorrow or do more exercise in the future. If you have avoided exercise and cutting calories for years, why would you expect it would be any different tomorrow?

Instead of giving yourself the license to head in the wrong direction, go in the right direction while you've got this book in front of you and the will to move forward.

SLIM FOR LIFE SECRET #18
Adopt a New Attitude

Have you ever noticed how whenever you complain, you feel even worse afterward? I have. I do it and then lament the time lost and the fact that I may have pulled someone else's mood down along with mine. Complaining can greatly impair your diet and exercise program results.

I often hear people say, "I'm not sure how much longer I can stand this stupid diet" or "I'm sweating like a pig at the gym every day and for what?" or "I hate to exercise" or "I hate to sweat." This kind of negative chatter — out loud or even allowed to run free inside your mind—gives you close to a zero percent chance of succeeding.

In the August 9, 2009 edition of *TIME*, in an article entitled "Why Exercise Won't Make You Thin," author John Cloud moans that his trainer "will work him like a farm animal, sometimes to the point that I am dizzy."

What exactly does this mean? That his trainer collared him, hooked a plow up to him and took him out to till the fields of New York City (do they even have fields there)? And men say that women are drama queens—Ha!

Anyway, back to my original point. If you say, "I hate it," you will hate it. If you say, "I can't do it," you won't succeed. Your mind really does govern your experience.

Here's an experiment you can try, which can give you some perspective on the mental aspect of experience. Frown for 20 minutes. Now pause to notice what kind of mood you are in. Now smile for 20 minutes and see what kind of mood you are in at this point. Now think about a place you really hate for five minutes. How do you feel? And now think of a place that is a peaceful sanctuary for you. Is your mood different? Attitude really is everything.

If you hate to sweat, remind yourself that you are ridding your body of toxins and making your fat cells cry. This is much more positive than whining. Your attitude will have more influence on whether you succeed at making positive changes than anything else in this book!

If you find a reason to love what you're doing for yourself, eventually it will become a comfortable part of your life. To me, my daily exercise is every bit as comforting to me as my 10-year-old pair of slippers and my afternoon cup of green tea. It is something I can depend on amidst life's many uncertainties.

Some ways to view this program (and to explain what you are doing to family and friends). "I'll feel so much better after I work out." "This class always helps me manage stress." "I feel empowered making good choices." "I'm making my body healthier." "I feel 20 years younger now that I'm taking better care of myself." "I'm not on a diet. I'm eating healthy foods that give me more energy, keep me satisfied, and taste better the more often I eat them."

You can even use these as mantras whenever you need a stress break and say one that speaks to you while you close your eyes and take a few deep breaths.

SLIM FOR LIFE SECRET #19
Live Young

When a woman's attitude ages, she may convince herself that she is too old to [fill in the blank] — watch what she eats, compete in athletic events, spend time exercising, wear shorts, bathing suits, bike pants and/or Spandex, or swim. And for that reason, she stops doing these things and before long the appearance of her body starts to match her mindset.

Just say "no" to that confining realm of thinking. Go ahead and buy the neon-colored tights or the thong bathing suit. And when your daughter asks you if you'd like to give her extra paddleboard a try, don the safety vest, grab a paddle and head out with her on a new adventure!

Before I met my husband and tried a dating service, I met a man who said on the phone he enjoyed cycling, hiking, rock climbing and scuba diving. I looked forward to meeting him and imagined all the outdoor adventures we would enjoy together.

When I met him, he confessed that he no longer did those activities. Now he was tired and busy with work and starting to have aches and pains. He was only in his mid 30s! That connection didn't last long.

I find it exhausting to spend time with people who act and think old. When I encountered them as clients, I tried to help them reframe their thinking so they could enjoy life more!

If you've given up activities you love for committees, shopping trips, TV, knitting, and other activities you somehow deem age appropriate, I suggest you reevaluate your priorities and mentally turn back the clock. If you're doing exercise that "people your age" do, rebel and try something fun instead. When was the last time you saw a child on a treadmill?

Just because you're over fifty doesn't mean you shouldn't have fun being active! If you love riding a unicycle (and have good bone density and excellent balance), go buy one. If you once loved trampolining (I do), purchase a big one or a mini-tramp, but make sure there are spotters all around you or that you have a safety net (or bar for the mini-tramp). Do you like horseback riding? Find a facility with well-trained horses where you can embark on a guided trail ride.

Reclaim your youthful perspective on exercise and you'll find it so much easier to be active.

I've studied the habits of many very fit older adults and their workout schedules and attire closely resemble those of people half their age.

They don't use their age as an excuse to be sedentary or to justify carrying around excess weight. They're not embarrassed to wear a swimsuit because of droopy skin or a few wrinkles. They continue to live the active lives they've always lived.

For me, the title of Olympic swimmer Dara Torres' book *Age is Just a Number* says it all. Shrug your shoulders and keep moving and you'll look a whole lot better than if you start telling yourself you're too old to do this or that anymore.

In 2008, I interviewed 90-year-old Rita Simonton, who set several world records for 90-94-year-old women at the U.S. Masters Long Course Swimming Nationals event in Portland, Oregon. When I punched in her number and waited for her to answer, I wondered if she might be easily confused or have trouble hearing. Instead, she was enthusiastic and quick-witted. Within minutes, I nearly forgot I was speaking to someone twice my age. She quickly showed her mind to be as agile as her body.

When training clients at SaddleBrooke, an active adult community in northwest Tucson, I saw the same familiar faces nearly every morning. Women in their 50s, 60s and even their 90s, clad in running shorts, Spandex bottoms, and/or tank tops that showed-off well-toned muscles.

They do Zumba classes, high intensity interval training (HIIT) workouts, strength training workouts, or core work and then head out to play tennis or golf. Some are on the community swimming team or members of the cycling or the hiking club. None of these people would say they are too old to go cycling or wear shorts or a form-fitting top.

One couple in their 80s came to the gym three times a week (in their cycling shorts after a ride) to lift weights together. Nancy always stood out from the crowd in her bright red cycling shorts!

I remember how she and Fred always took turns spotting each other on the bench press machine. There's something about seeing couples support each other in their training efforts that always warms my heart.

In Mexico, I have a friend in her mid-70s who mountain bikes for two to three hours more than once a week. She broke a forearm bone once, but that didn't stop her from getting back to it once the doctor cleared her to! Mountain biking is what she enjoys most and so she continues to pursue it with passion!

Many other friends and neighbors in their 70s are out kayaking with the dolphins most days of the week (there are "pedal" kayaks available on the market today that don't require upper body strength and work better for people with previous shoulder issues). My neighbors recently bought stair-stepper style paddleboards that look like a blast to move around on.

Stock up on shoes and other athletic wear that you will need to move comfortably when exercising. Consider leaving the gray and black workout wear on the rack and step out in something bright and flashy that you imagine area high school kids would envy. If it makes you feel excited about what you are about to do, why not go for it?

SLIM FOR LIFE SECRET #20
Drink Water Before You Eat

Most of us have heard that worn-out suggestion to drink water before each meal. That's a good tip to remember anytime you feel hungry. Sometimes signals get crossed and you feel hungry when you're really dehydrated.

When a snack attack strikes, drink a glass of water before opening the refrigerator. Often the water will provide a sense of fullness and you'll consume less food as a result.

Consuming water improves digestion and increases metabolism. Always drink a glass of water before your breakfast, lunch, and dinner.

A study showed that dieters drinking 500 ml of water (16.9 ounces) before meals experienced more weight loss than the people restricting calorie consumption who didn't consume the pre-meal water.

SLIM FOR LIFE SECRET #21
Jump-Start Metabolism with EPOC

Excess post-exercise oxygen consumption (EPOC) sounds like a phrase for scientists. That's true, but what this "after burn" means for you is that if you do the right workouts, you can burn beaucoup calories even after your workout ends. Your resting metabolic rate will be higher all day, which will make it easier for you to lose weight!

After strenuous activity, your body continues to consume more oxygen (the way it does during activity) to restore balance in the body's systems (digestion, cellular activity, muscle repair, etc.). The caloric burning is higher immediately post-exercise and gradually begins to taper off.

High- intensity interval cardio workouts (HIIT) and long duration workouts have been shown to incite the highest EPOC levels.

Your interval workouts don't have to be super complicated. You can run (outside or on the treadmill) for a minute and then walk for a minute to recover and continue with similar or different intervals. If you're a swimmer, after warming up, you can propel yourself through some sprint 50s with a rest interval in between. Or you can don an Aqua Jogger vest and run suspended intervals of fast running for 30-45 seconds with 15 seconds rest in between.

Whether you're training on land or in the water, music can be a helpful motivator. Music listening products you can use in the water are available at swimoutlet.com.

SLIM FOR LIFE SECRET #22
Fidget Your Weight Off with NEAT

Maybe you know someone thin who never sits still. She's always in motion, waving her hands when she speaks, jumping up and down when she's excited, running off for another game of tennis or softball or golf.

They're the ones we want to hate — they appear to eat whatever they want and never gain a pound. But their secret to leanness is available to you and everyone else. Beyond the psychology of why we sometimes make poor diet and exercise choices, weight loss primarily boils down to getting the body to burn or utilize more calories than are consumed. That thick slice of pie or handful of Doritos you see that annoying thin woman eating in the break room will be burned off in no time, because tennis burns calories, as does pacing and flailing your arms all over the place.

Mayo Clinic studies show that the number of calories a person burns during activities of daily living, also known as non-exercise activity thermogenesis (NEAT), affects a person's tendency to convert excess calories to fat.

A study following 20 individuals showed that the obese individuals spent an average of 164 minutes more per day sitting than the lean participants. Lean individuals also burned nearly 365 NEAT calories per day, which translates to a 36.5-pound weight loss in one year.

What this means to you is that a little fidgeting here and a little pacing the room there can make a tremendous difference in your weight over time.

This doesn't mean you should toss your gym shoes in the recesses of your closet. Regular exercise is crucial to your emotional, cardiovascular, muscular and bone health as well as an effective way to burn calories and keep metabolism high. But what you do in between your workouts is as important as what you do during them.

To take full advantage of NEAT, try the following:

1 - If you don't need to sit, stand instead. You burn more calories standing than sitting. If it isn't necessary to lie down, sit up instead. You burn more calories sitting than reclined. Sitting for long periods of time is as harmful for your health as it is for your waistline.

2 – Walk while standing when possible (when talking on the phone, for example). Pace around, assemble or fix something, dust furniture or fold laundry when you talk.

3 – When shopping, instead of driving around for 10 minutes looking for a parking spot, park in a vacant spot further from the store.

4 – Take short walks after lunch or dinner. When waiting for a meeting or appointment, walk up and down the halls instead of dropping into a chair.

5 – Do your own cleaning and gardening whenever possible.

6 – Pursue active hobbies such as golf, bird watching, walking, kayaking, tennis, hiking, playing a musical instrument (standing), and swimming.

7 – If you must watch television, stretch, or exercise on the stability ball during part of the program. Or instead of reclining, sit up.

8 – Use your hands when you speak—it will hold people's attention and burn more calories.

9 – If the fitness facility, luncheon, or other event is within walking distance, leave your car at home and head out on foot instead.

SLIM FOR LIFE SECRET #23
Stay in Places with a Kitchen When Traveling

Most people assume they'll gain weight when travelling. Pancake breakfasts, burgers grabbed on the go for lunch, and steak and shrimp dinners served with bottles of wine. There's no doubt that all these meals out can be hazardous to your weight. So why not implement my secret weapon to combat this?

My husband and I travel often — not only in the U.S. but to many other countries. And we've found it super helpful to take our own (allowed) healthy snacks in our check-in luggage and reserve rentals with a kitchen. With Airbnb so popular, it's easy to find a place where you can prepare your own meals, not to mention that many of these apartments and condos often are much more comfortable than hotels.

Ask in advance what's in the kitchen at the rental so the owner can buy additional items you need in advance. Even if you do have to go out and buy a cheese grater or a decent paring knife after you arrive, you'll still save money eating in instead of dining out every meal. And you'll have more time for site-seeing since you won't be spending so much time waiting to get a table or for food to be served.

SLIM FOR LIFE SECRET #24
Use Competition as a Motivational Carrot

Competition isn't for everyone, but for many people it can provide motivation to keep exercising or step it up another notch. It's another form of goal setting. People of all ages can race. Athletes more mature than 80 compete in running events, cycling races, swim meets and triathlons — accumulating medals and trophies that make their friends envious. Most active adult communities offer tennis and golf tournaments and some even have competitive softball and soccer.

If you have a competitive streak in you, use it to your advantage. When I joined U.S. Masters Swimming and started racing, I dragged myself out of bed for 6 AM practice more often than I would have had I been swimming laps on my own.

What if you've never competed before or you don't consider yourself athletic? Does that mean you should never turn out for a 5K run or walkathon? Definitely not.

Once you participate in an event, you will see that people show up with many different objectives. The myth of athletic competitions is that every participant is skinny, wears revealing clothing and runs a 6- minute mile. Not true. As a matter of fact, at the events I have competed in, most of the competitors carried a few extra pounds and most finished in times that would be considered closer to a walking than a running pace. And they still had a great time!

Don't allow your ego to get in the way of enjoying yourself. It doesn't matter whether you're slow or fast. Just getting out and participating is an achievement. I'm not the best runner, but I push myself harder with a group than if I'm running around the block alone.

Even if I don't cross the finish line lightning fast, I always finish knowing I got a great workout and — on top of that — I feel energized and upbeat for the rest of the day. These benefits more than compensate for any "embarrassment" I might experience due to my lack of running ability. I'm far more skilled at swimming, but that's okay.

Since my husband and I participate in many athletic events together and swimming isn't his forte (unlike me, he's a skilled runner), we each sign up for races in our weaker sports.

Many of my former clients in the active adult community of SaddleBrooke (in northwest Tucson) play competitive tennis or pickleball, compete in swimming races, or do triathlons. If you live in a similar community, most likely the HOA hosts a website that lists groups and training times.

The people I know at SaddleBrooke are invigorated by the camaraderie, motivating atmosphere and excitement of competition (even those pre-race jitters and talking with others about them can be fun).

Competitive events come in all types. The most common include running events, walking or run/walk events, and cycling events. You can find U.S. Masters Swimming teams and competitions for pool and open water in your area at usms.org. U.S. Masters Swimming offers local and national competitions in most major U.S. cities. Groups such as Everyone Runs and Southern Arizona Roadrunners offer running races in the Tucson area. Perimeter Bicycling offers cycling events in southern Arizona.

Almost anyone who works out 30 minutes three or more days a week can finish a 5K run or a charity walk or even a short bicycling event. The trick is to find an event that suits your interests and abilities. If you can't swim more than one length of the pool without stopping, the triathlon isn't for you. However, if you've been stuck in a training rut and know how to swim, cycle and run, mixing up your training with these three activities can be fun.

Crossing training enables you to work more muscles over the course of your training week and reduces your potential for injury. You can rest your upper body on non-swimming days and your knees and ankles on days you take to the water instead of running. Working a variety of muscles with these different training modalities can deliver an amazing looking physique.

If the word "triathlon" brings the word "Ironman" to mind, think again. Triathlons come in all shapes and sizes. The sprint triathlon is accessible to most fit individuals and, although distances vary, usually involves an 800-yard swim, a 12-mile bike ride and a 3-mile run.

Some events offer relays where you can team up with two friends or family members and each of you do one segment of the race.

I've competed in dozens of sprint triathlons over the years. If you prefer lake or ocean over pool swimming, there are many open water events available. The U.S. Masters Swimming site lists pool and open water events. I've competed in open water races in Arizona (https://www.azopenwaterseries.com), La Jolla, CA (https://thelajollacoveswim.org/), Bellingham, WA (https://globalswimseries.com/aly-fell-open-water-swim/) and Guaymas and Kino Bay, Mexico.

If you prefer mountain biking and trail running over hitting the pavement, you can give an X-Terra event a go. Many events for different endurance sports can be found at http://www.active.com.

SLIM FOR LIFE SECRET #25
Derive Inspiration from a Role Model

Often when I'm working toward a goal, I try to emulate the behavior of a successful person I admire. Some of my favorite role models are Al Jarreau (for his zest for life and amazing creativity; sadly he passed away on February 12, 2017), Michael Phelps and Dara Torres (for Olympic swimming and their amazing bodies) and Stephen King and Nicholas Sparks (for their discipline and writing achievements).

Stephen King's *On Writing* not only gave me a great deal of insight into King as a person, but outlined the writing habits that enable him to produce a tremendous amount of publishable work.

Watching Michael Phelps and Dara Torres swim in the 2008 Beijing Olympics fueled my desire to train harder. I was in awe when Phelps made a comeback and showed off his winning ways again in 2012 and 2016.

At age 54, Dara Torres has a leaner, fitter body than most women half her age. She was 41 when she competed in her last Olympics. Activity is as much a mantra for Dara (I've given myself creative license to refer to my heroes on a first name basis) as it is for me.

Even when Dara took a hiatus from competitive swimming, she remained active. In addition to daily swim workouts, when she prepared for the 2008 Olympics, she poured her heart into strength training, core work, and stretching.

It thrilled me to hear she'd qualified for the 2008 Olympics and on a big screen after a day of racing at the U.S. Masters Swimming Long Course Nationals in Portland, I watched Dara win a silver medal in the 50-meter freestyle in Beijing. Reading about her and watching her compete in the Olympics inspired me to reach my 2008 Long Course Masters swimming goals.

As a matter of fact, I was so inspired that I obtained three personal best swimming times at the Masters Summer Nationals Swimming Championship, placing 2nd in the 100 and 200-meter breaststroke and 3rd in the 50-meter breaststroke.

Al Jarreau has been my favorite musician since I was 20. Listening to his familiar voice and his upbeat music has pulled me through some very difficult times. The optimism in his music always inspired me to live happy and to express joy and positive energy. I attended two of his concerts — exhilarating experiences both times. There is something about his energy that was so uplifting.

The second one of Al's concerts I attended in Scottsdale was less than a month before he passed away. Despite chronic back pain and other health difficulties and the need to lean on a stool for support, he delivered an amazing performance. He kept on touring the world, doing what he loved up until the very end. Music, performing, and uplifting others were his reason for living.

The more I know about how other successful people work and live, the easier it is to construct my own strategy for achievement. During times of difficulty, I often think, "How would my hero/heroine handle this?" Emulating positive behaviors and lifestyles helps you get closer to obtaining the healthy and fitter body you've always wanted to have!

So how can my role models help you? I hope that you'll develop a burning desire to push yourself harder and achieve goals you might otherwise not achieve by emulating people you admire and can identify with. Look for people who are living a healthy lifestyle and that will inspire you reach your fitness, weight, and nutrition goals. If you read about their lives and how they achieved goals, you will find yourself wanting to emulate them.

I'll never win an Olympic gold, of that, I'm sure. But I can continue to swim my personal bests, just as Dara Torres has done. And why is that? Largely because I believe it is possible. Reading articles about her in *Swimming World* and *Sports Illustrated* and watching her swim on TV kept me excited and motivated.

I see some of her in myself. I'm a mom, too. I have a busy schedule. I do lots of cross training. I have been active all my life. And I'm swimming personal bests. We have a whole lot in common, and I feel her energy with me whenever I'm pushing myself.

Dara stays slim because the number of calories she burns in daily activities is equivalent to the calories she puts back into her body. The end result? At the end of the day, no excess calories are stored as pounds of fat on her midsection.

I've heard younger swimmers muse about how odd it is that Dara still trains hard at her age, as if after a certain age, one should slip into a comfortable sedentary state, parking oneself in front of the television with a beer and a bowl of potato chips.

I admire Dara for her efforts and achievements — she has decided that staying in top physical condition is something she will do, not for a few years until she medals at the Olympics or wins the college conference championships, but for life.

I happen to be a very athletic person and so athletes provide a lot of fuel for my fire. Not all of you will find an athlete to be an appropriate role model. Choose someone who represents what you want to become. It could be your neighbor who walks three miles religiously every morning before work or a movie star who manages to stay fit and trim despite a hectic filming schedule.

SLIM FOR LIFE SECRET #26
Confront the Saboteurs

You've heard about people who deep-six the diets of loved ones. Maybe you find it hard to believe anyone would behave like that. Why would anyone want a spouse, daughter, sister, or friend to fail at efforts to improve health? The answer is complicated.

Maybe your spouse isn't ready to change his or her eating habits. Maybe he's worried you will encourage him to eat smaller portions or reduce the amount of fat in his diet (he won't like it one bit if you identify his peanut-eating during the ballgame as "mindless"). A person feels more comfortable engaging in poor lifestyle choices when around "comforting" relatives and friends making the same mistakes. The dieter is about as much fun to a group of over-eaters as the teetotaler is to the bar crowd.

You may still be a little afraid of the changes you're making. But you have had time to ponder them and to decide a healthy lifestyle is what you want.

Some of your family and friends may be afraid of your new habits and not be ready to make a commitment to positive changes. They may worry what you're doing will make them feel guilty for sticking with the status quo or that you might become a different person if you lose weight.

Ideally, you can persuade the saboteur to overcome his or her insecurities and adopt healthier habits. In the real world, you will have to explain your expectations. Tell your spouse or friend there are wellness goals you want to accomplish and that you don't have any expectations for them to change, but that you expect support for your efforts. If the person continues to encourage you to overeat or to miss exercise sessions, stand your ground! Don't cave in.

Explain the importance of what you are doing and how this new lifestyle is important to your health and is now part of your identity. If the person really loves you, he or she will eventually come around.

SLIM FOR LIFE SECRET #27
Add Mung Beans to Your Diet

Most people unfamiliar with Ayurveda have never heard of mung beans, a legume in the same family as peas and lentils. Quite simply, they're packed with nutrients, reduce inflammation, and improve digestive health. I often use them in soups.

If time is of the essence, throwing a bunch of healthy ingredients in the crock-pot in the morning is a great way to return home after work to a meal already prepared!

You can also make kitchari, which is very healthy and easy to prepare. There are many different variations. Here is one way to prepare it.

Ingredients

2 cups yellow mung dal beans

2 tbsp ghee or organic sesame oil

2 tsp black mustard seeds

2 tsp cumin seeds

1 tsp fennel seeds

1 tsp fenugreek seeds

2 tsp ground turmeric

2 tsp ground black pepper

1 tsp ground cumin

1 tsp ground coriander

1 tsp cinnamon

1 cup uncooked white basmati rice

2–5 cups of chopped, organic, seasonal vegetables (spinach, carrots, beets, sweet potato, squash, celery, kale, and bok choy)

2 cloves

2 bay leaves

3 green cardamom pods

1 cup chopped fresh cilantro (optional)

Directions

Rinse and strain the mung dal beans until the water runs clear. In a large pot, heat the ghee or oil. Add the black mustard, cumin, fennel, and fenugreek seeds and toast until the mustard seeds pop. Add turmeric, black pepper, cumin, coriander, and cinnamon, and then mix them together.

Stir in the rice and beans. Add 8 cups of water, chopped vegetables, cloves, bay leaves, and cardamom pods. Bring to a boil and reduce to a simmer.

Cook at least one hour, until the beans and rice are soft and the kitchari has a porridge-like consistency. Serve warm with fresh cilantro on top, if desired.

Mung beans are rich in potassium, folate (Vitamin B9), Vitamin B1 and B6, magnesium, manganese, copper and zinc. They're also high in protein and dietary fiber, which give a feeling of satiety and reduce the temptation to overeat.

A study published in the *Journal of Nutrition* revealed that a single meal with high-fiber beans produced a two-fold greater increase in the satiety hormone called cholecystokinin when compared to meals that didn't contain beans.

Because mung beans are so nutrient-rich, they are considered protective against diabetes, cancer, heart disease and obesity. They can lower LDL (bad) cholesterol, reduce inflammation, and scavenge free radicals in the body that can damage DNA.

Mung beans have a high carbohydrate content and work well for making flour and noodle products. In Chinese cuisine, mung beans are used to make pancakes or dumplings, combined with rice in stir-fries, and used to make tángshuǐ, in which the beans are cooked with sugar, coconut milk and a pinch of ginger. After cooking they can also be stirred into hummus or other dips or pureed to thicken soups.

SLIM FOR LIFE SECRET #28
Don't Push Through the Wrong Kind of Pain

I've encouraged you to exercise often and even at a high intensity when it's appropriate. But sometimes when you exercise, you'll experience something worse than your heart rate elevating and simple muscle fatigue. Maybe you feel lightheaded or dizzy or confused. In these instances, you should immediately stop and if these symptoms don't quickly subside, you should call 9-1-1.

Sometimes you'll feel a strain in a muscle or joint during movement or feel pain in a joint such as the shoulder or hip. I've heard swimmers on our Masters swimming team say, "My shoulder hurts." Between sets they grimace and rub the sore area, but they force themselves to swim for another hour. Anytime I experience something similar, I slow my pace or stop.

When you feel muscle pain that doesn't subside immediately when you stop exercise (such as a burn in the muscles you feel during a strength training set), you're experiencing strain or repetitive stress injury. This is a cue from your body to stop.

The best way to keep this minor injury from turning into a major one is to rest that part of the body for two or three days and apply an ice pack on it regularly to reduce inflammation. Regular massages can help alleviate irregularities in connective tissue that can potentially cause pain.

It won't serve you well to push through the pain. It will only put you at risk for injury, which could lead to you being unable to exercise or requiring surgery.

One of the best ways to reduce injuries is to cross train. Engage in different activities throughout your week so you're not constantly over-using the same muscles and risking a repetitive stress injury.

Instead of swimming or running or cycling five days per week, swim on Tuesdays and Thursdays, run or walk on Mondays and Fridays, and cycle on Wednesdays and Saturdays (or assemble your own "different activities" combination)!

Always include low or non-impact activities (walking, swimming, elliptical, cycling) each week. Cross-training enables you to exercise more with much less wear and tear on your body.

SLIM FOR LIFE SECRET #29
Adopt a Dog

Research has shown that owning a dog enhances happiness, reduces anxiety, and improves overall mental health.

If you adopt a dog from a shelter, you may very well be saving his or her life. Adopting a furry friend is also guaranteed to get you up off that couch!

Your dog will depend on you for daily walks. Taking your pet out will be a responsibility as well as an opportunity to exercise, enhancing your adherence. You'll bond during these outdoor treks together and both of you will be getting fresh air, moving muscles, and elevating heart rate for better health.

SLIM FOR LIFE SECRET #30
After a Slip-Up, Jump Back on Track

If you get off track, jump back into the arena instead of continuing to binge or eat the wrong foods. Many people that deviate from a healthy eating program they've started figure "oh, well, I already messed up" and continue to overindulge for the rest of the day or even longer. Don't be one of these people!

Keep in mind that it takes an excess of 3500 calories to gain a pound, so if you slip up and eat two pieces of pie, you won't gain weight if you avoid overeating the rest of the day. Forgive and forget, rather than allowing yourself to tumble into an abyss of guilt and recrimination. If you get back on track quickly, you'll keep losing weight.

SLIM FOR LIFE SECRET #31
Lose for Health and for You

This journey to a healthier, slimmer you is all about you! Don't lose weight to look like a cover model or to please your family and friends.

Instead of trying to suit other peoples' concepts of what looks good (which usually leaves you feeling resentful and not wanting to do anything to change), set achievable goals that meet your desires and embark on a journey to move toward them.

If you need more resources to help you on your wellness journey, please consider reading *Fitter Than Ever at 40 and Beyond* or *Fitter Than*

Ever at 50 and Beyond. These books include detailed information on starting an exercise program (and avoiding injuries), diet and nutrition, mindful living, and much more. I also post many motivating articles and tips on my blog that you might find helpful at https://www.fitwomenrock.com

REFERENCES/RECOMMENDED READING

An, R. 2016. "Beverage Consumption in Relation to Discretionary Food Intake and Diet Quality among US Adults, 2003 to 2012." *Journal of the Academy of Nutrition and Dietetics.* 116(1):28-37.

Balch, P. 2010. *Prescription for Nutritional Healing Fifth Edition: A Practical A-to-Z Reference to Drug-Free Remedies Using Vitamins, Herbs, and Food Supplements.* New York: Avery (a member of Penguin Group).

Borsheim, E., and R. Bahr. 2003. "Effect of Exercise, Intensity, Duration and Mode on Post-Exercise Oxygen Consumption." *Sports Medicine.* 33(14): 1037-60.

Boschmann, M. 2003. "Water-induced thermogenesis." *Journal of Clinical Endocrinology and Metabolism,* 12(88), 6015-6019.

Comana, F. 2012. The Energy Balance Equation. *IDEA Fitness Journal.* 9(3).

Center for Science in the Public Interest. 2013. "CSPI Downgrades Splenda from 'Safe' to 'Caution.'" https://cspinet.org/new/201306121.html

Chow, L., E. Manoogian, A. Alvear, J. Fleischer, H. Thor, K. Dietsche, Q. Wang, J. Hodges, N. Esch, S. Malaeb, T. Harindhanavudhi, K. Nair, S. Panda, and D. Mashek. 2020. "Time Restricted Eating Effects on Body Composition and Metabolic Measures in Humans Who are Overweight: A Feasibility Study." *Obesity.* 28(5): 860-869.

Cox, L. 2012. "Why is Too Much Salt Bad for You?" *Live Science online* (http://www.livescience.com/36256-salt-bad-health.html)

Dennis E.A., A.L. Dengo, D.L. Comber, K.D. Flack, J. Savla, K.P. Davy, and B.M. Davy. 2010. "Water consumption increases weight loss during a hypocaloric diet intervention in middle-aged and older adults." *Obesity, 18*(2), 300-7.

Ford, H.E., V. Peters, N.M. Martin, M.L. Sleeth, M.A. Ghatei, G.S. Frost, and S.R. Bloom. 2011. "Effects of oral ingestion of sucralose on gut hormone response and appetite in healthy normal-weight subjects." *European Journal of Clinical Nutrition.* 65 (4): 508–13.

Grattan, B.J., Jr., and J. Connolly-Schoonen, J. 2012. "Addressing weight loss recidivism: a clinical focus on metabolic rate and the psychological aspects of obesity." *ISRN Obesity.* 2012: 567530.

Hall, J., S.M. Skevington, P.J. Maddison, and K. Chapman. 1996. "A randomized and controlled trial of hydrotherapy in rheumatoid arthritis." *Arthritis Care Research,* 9(3): 206-215.

Halvorson, R. 2015. "Frequent Sitting Means Weight Gain for Women." *IDEA Fitness Journal.* 12(3).

Hill, A.J. 2004. "Does dieting make you fat?" *British Journal of Nutrition, 92*(1), S5–S18.

Ingeborg, B., B. Olson, R. Backus, D. Richter, P. Davis, and B. Schneeman. (2001). "Beans, as a Source of Dietary Fiber, Increase Cholecystokinin and Apolipoprotein B48

Response to Test Meals in Men." *Journal of Nutrition.* 131: 1485-1490.

Kolata, G. 2016. "After 'The Biggest Loser' Their Bodies Fought to Regain the Weight." *The Science of Fat.* (NY Times online post) https://www.nytimes.com/2016/05/02/health/biggest-loser-weight-loss.html)

Kravitz, L. 2006. "A NEAT 'new' strategy for weight control." *IDEA Fitness Journal*, 3(4), 24-25.

Kravitz, L. 2009. "Calorie burning: It's time to think 'outside the box.'" *IDEA Fitness Journal*, 6(4), 32-38.

Lee, I.M., L. Djoussé, H.D. Sesso, L. Wang, and J.E. Buring. 2010. "Physical activity and weight gain prevention." *JAMA.* 303(12):1173-1179.

Levitt, A.J. 2005. *The Kripalu Cookbook: Gourmet Vegetarian Recipes.* Countryman Press.

Manini, T.M. 2010. "Energy expenditure and aging." *Ageing Research Reviews.* 9(1): 1-11.

Matthews, M. Muscle for Life https://www.muscleforlife.com/tdee-calculator/

McArdle, W., R. Glasner, and J. Magel. 1971. "Metabolic and cardio-respiratory responses during free swimming and treadmill walking." *Journal of Applied Physiology*. 33(5): 733-738.

McMurray, R.G., J. Soares, C.J. Casperson, and T. McCurdy. 2014. "Examining variations of resting metabolic rate of adults: a public health perspective." *Medicine and Sciences in Sports and Exercise*. 46 (7): 1352-1358.

National Heart, Blood, and Lung Institute https://www.nhlbi.nih.gov/health/education al/lose_wt/BMI/bmi_tbl.htm

O'Donnell, K. (Author) and C. Brostrom (Photographer). 2015. *The Everyday Ayerveda Cookbook: A Seasonal Guide to Eating and Living Well*. Boulder, CO: Shambhala Publications, Inc.

Parker-Pope, T. 2009. "How the Food Makers Captured Our Brains." *New York Times online*. (http://www.nytimes.com/2009/06/23/healt h/23well.html)

Peeke, P. 2012. "The Dopamine Made Me Do it." *IDEA Fitness Journal*. 9(9): 34-42.

Prochaska, J.O., J.C. Norcross, and C.C. DiClemente. 1994. *Changing For Good: The Revolutionary Program That Explains The Six*

Stages Of Change And Teaches You How To Free Yourself From Bad Habits. New York: W. Morrow.

Rabin, R. 2016. "Artificial Sweeteners and Weight Gain." New York Times Blog. https://well.blogs.nytimes.com/2016/02/19/artificial-sweeteners-and-weight-gain/

Sutton E.F., R. Beyl, K.S. Early, W.T. Cefalu, E. Ravussin, and C.M. Peterson. 2018. "Early Time-Restricted Feeding Improves Insulin Sensitivity, Blood Pressure, and Oxidative Stress Even without Weight Loss in Men with Prediabetes." *Cell Metabolism* 27(6): 1212–1221.e3.

Tirrito, S. 2009. *So You're Fat. Now What?* Wheatmark.

Truth in Labeling. http://www.truthinlabeling.org/hiddensources.html

Wilkinson M., E. Manoogian, A. Zadourian, H. Lo, S. Fakhouri, A. Shoghi, X. Wang, J. Fleisher, S Navlakha, S. Panda, and P. Taub. 2020. "Ten-Hour Time-Restricted Eating Reduces Weight, Blood Pressure, and Atherogenic Lipids in Patients with Metabolic Syndrome." *Cell Metabolism* 31(1): 92–104.e105.

Wyatt, F.B., S. Milam, R.C. Manske, and R. Deere. 2001. "The effects of aquatic and traditional exercise programs on persons with knee osteoarthritis," *Journal of Strength Conditioning Research*, 15(3): 337-340.

Printed in Great Britain
by Amazon